Table Of Contents

Chapter 1: Introduction to the Carnivore Diet

What is the Carnivore Diet?

The Carnivore Diet, often described as a meat-based dietary regimen, revolves around the exclusive consumption of animal products. This approach eliminates all plant-based foods, focusing solely on meat, fish, eggs, and dairy (for those who tolerate it). The simplicity of the diet is one of its most appealing aspects, as it removes the complexities of calorie counting, meal prepping with varied ingredients, and the need for extensive meal planning. For many, the Carnivore Diet offers an enticing path to weight loss, thanks to its high protein content and potential to promote satiety, which can lead to reduced overall caloric intake.

At its core, the Carnivore Diet is built on the premise that humans can thrive on an animal-based diet. Proponents argue that our ancestors primarily consumed meat, and modern dietary guidelines have strayed too far from this natural inclination. Supporters claim that the diet can lead to numerous health benefits, including weight loss, improved mental clarity, and better digestion. However, as with any dietary approach, it is crucial to consider individual health needs and consult with healthcare professionals before making significant changes.

For beginners, transitioning to the Carnivore Diet can be a daunting task, especially when faced with the elimination of familiar foods. However, understanding the basics of the diet can ease this transition. Start by stocking up on a variety of meats, such as beef, chicken, pork, and fish, as well as eggs and cheese for those who include dairy. Planning meals around these staples can help establish a routine, and as your palate adjusts, you may find yourself appreciating the flavors and textures of different cuts of meat. Budget-conscious individuals can explore local butcher shops, farmers' markets, and sales at grocery stores to find high-quality meat options at lower prices.

Challenges may arise during the initial phase of adopting the Carnivore Diet, including cravings for carbohydrates and the social implications of dining out or attending events. Preparing for these challenges can make the transition smoother. Consider meal prepping in advance, so you always have a nutritious option readily available. Additionally, learning to navigate menus at restaurants can provide opportunities to enjoy social gatherings without compromising dietary goals. Emphasizing the importance of community support, whether through online forums or local groups, can also provide motivation and accountability.

Ultimately, the Carnivore Diet presents an intriguing option for those seeking weight loss and a simplified approach to nutrition. By embracing the principles of this diet, individuals may discover newfound energy, satisfaction, and clarity in their eating habits. Understanding the strategies for maintaining a meat-based diet on a budget, as well as the potential challenges and solutions for beginners, will empower readers to confidently embark on their journey. As with any lifestyle change, patience and perseverance are key, and with time, the rewards of the Carnivore Diet may become increasingly apparent.

Benefits of a Meat-Based Diet

A meat-based diet, particularly the carnivore diet, has gained attention for its potential health benefits, especially for individuals seeking weight loss. One of the most significant advantages of a carnivore diet is its simplicity and focus on whole, unprocessed foods. By eliminating carbohydrates and sugars, the body is encouraged to enter a state of ketosis, where it burns fat for fuel instead of relying on glucose. This metabolic shift can lead to effective weight loss, as individuals may find it easier to manage hunger and cravings when consuming nutrient-dense animal products.

Another benefit of a meat-based diet is its ability to promote satiety. Protein is known for its satiating properties, and meals centered around meat can help individuals feel fuller for longer periods. This can reduce the frequency of snacking and ultimately lead to a lower overall caloric intake. For those on a budget, focusing on protein-rich foods such as beef, chicken, and pork can provide substantial nutrition without the need for expensive, processed weight loss products. By prioritizing meat, individuals can achieve their weight loss goals while remaining mindful of their finances.

Additionally, a carnivore diet can simplify meal planning and preparation, making it an attractive option for beginners. With fewer food choices, individuals can streamline their grocery lists and meal prep routines, minimizing the time and effort spent on cooking and shopping. This can be particularly beneficial for those who may feel overwhelmed by the complexity of traditional dieting methods that require extensive meal planning. By sticking to meat and animal-based products, newcomers can quickly familiarize themselves with the essentials of the diet, paving the way for a smoother transition.

The carnivore diet also affords potential health benefits beyond weight loss, which can be motivating factors for individuals embarking on this dietary journey. Many adherents report improvements in energy levels, mental clarity, and digestive health. The elimination of processed foods and sugars can lead to reduced inflammation and better overall well-being. As individuals experience these positive changes, it can reinforce their commitment to the diet, further supporting weight loss goals and promoting a healthier lifestyle.

Finally, embracing a meat-based diet does not have to be a financial burden. There are various strategies for maintaining a carnivore lifestyle on a budget, such as buying in bulk, selecting less expensive cuts of meat, and utilizing seasonal sales. By planning meals around sales and utilizing resources like local farmers or butcher shops, individuals can enjoy the benefits of a meat-based diet without overspending. This adaptability makes the carnivore diet an accessible option for those looking to lose weight while adhering to financial constraints.

Understanding the Science Behind Carnivorism

Understanding the science behind carnivorism is essential for anyone considering the carnivore diet, especially those looking to manage their weight effectively while keeping costs down. At its core, the carnivore diet consists entirely of animal-based foods, emphasizing meat, fish, and animal-derived products. This approach challenges conventional dietary guidelines that advocate for a more plant-based intake. By delving into the biochemical and physiological principles at play, we can better appreciate how this diet impacts weight loss, metabolic health, and overall well-being.

One of the primary mechanisms through which the carnivore diet influences weight loss is its effect on insulin levels. Consuming a diet devoid of carbohydrates leads to lower insulin production, a hormone that plays a significant role in fat storage. When insulin levels drop, the body begins to utilize stored fat for energy, facilitating weight loss. Additionally, high protein intake from meat helps promote satiety, which can reduce overall calorie consumption. Understanding these hormonal responses can empower beginners to make informed choices about their food intake and portion sizes while following a budget-friendly approach.

Another important aspect of the carnivore diet is its impact on nutrient density. Animal products are rich in essential nutrients such as vitamins B12, iron, and omega-3 fatty acids, which are often lacking in plant-based diets. For those on a budget, focusing on high-quality cuts of meat and organ meats can provide a cost-effective way to ensure adequate nutrition. This nutrient density is not only critical for maintaining energy levels but also supports the body's metabolic processes, promoting efficient weight loss. Learning how to source these ingredients affordably can help beginners adhere to this diet without overspending.

The science of adaptation is also crucial for understanding the carnivore diet. When transitioning to a meat-based diet, individuals may initially experience a period of adjustment where the body shifts from burning carbohydrates to utilizing fat as its primary fuel source. This metabolic shift, often referred to as ketosis, can lead to increased fat oxidation and weight loss. However, it is essential to approach this transition thoughtfully, incorporating strategies to ease the process, such as gradually reducing carbohydrate intake and staying well-hydrated. This can help mitigate potential challenges, such as fatigue or digestive discomfort, that may arise during the initial stages.

Lastly, understanding the psychological and behavioral aspects of eating is vital for success on the carnivore diet. Many individuals struggle with cravings and food habits shaped by societal norms and marketing. By recognizing the role of meat as a satiating and nutrient-rich food source, dieters can cultivate a positive relationship with their meals. Strategies such as meal planning, batch cooking, and seeking out budget-friendly meat options can further support adherence to the carnivore diet. By equipping themselves with knowledge about the science behind carnivorism, beginners can navigate their weight loss journey with confidence, ultimately making informed, health-conscious choices that align with their financial goals.

Chapter 2: Getting Started

Assessing Your Current Diet

Assessing your current diet is a crucial first step in transitioning to the carnivore diet, especially when weight loss is your primary goal. Understanding what you currently consume allows you to identify patterns, habits, and potential areas for improvement. Start by keeping a detailed food journal for at least one week, documenting everything you eat and drink. Note portion sizes, meal timings, and how you feel after each meal. This exercise will help you recognize not only the types of foods you are eating but also the emotional and psychological triggers that may influence your choices.

As you review your food journal, pay close attention to the macronutrient composition of your meals. The carnivore diet primarily consists of animal products, which means you'll be shifting away from carbohydrates and possibly some fats and proteins found in plant-based foods. Analyze your current intake of carbohydrates, sugars, and processed foods. Understanding where these elements fit into your diet will help you make more informed decisions as you move toward a meat-based regimen. Aim to reduce your reliance on high-carb foods to prepare your body for the transition, making it easier to adopt the carnivore diet effectively.

Another important aspect of assessing your current diet is evaluating your budget. Many newcomers to the carnivore diet worry about the costs associated with purchasing high-quality meats. Examine your current grocery spending and identify areas where you can cut back on non-essential items. Consider the trade-offs involved in prioritizing meat over processed foods or takeout meals. By reallocating your budget, you can create a sustainable plan that allows you to enjoy the health benefits of the carnivore diet without straining your finances. Look for sales, local butchers, and bulk purchasing options to maximize your savings.

In addition to financial considerations, reflect on your current health status and weight loss goals. Are there specific health issues or weight challenges that motivate your interest in the carnivore diet? Understanding your personal motivations can provide clarity and reinforce your commitment during the transition. Consult with a healthcare professional or nutritionist if necessary, especially if you have pre-existing conditions. They can help you assess the potential benefits of the carnivore diet in relation to your specific health needs and offer tailored advice for your journey.

Finally, as you assess your current diet, keep in mind the psychological aspects of changing eating habits. Transitioning to a carnivore diet can be a significant lifestyle shift, and it's normal to experience challenges along the way. Prepare yourself mentally by setting realistic expectations and acknowledging that change takes time. Embrace the journey with an open mind, and be ready to adapt your approach as you learn what works best for your body and budget. By thoroughly assessing your current diet, you'll be well-equipped to embark on your carnivore journey with confidence and clarity.

Setting Realistic Goals

Setting realistic goals is a fundamental aspect of embarking on any dietary journey, particularly when transitioning to the carnivore diet. This approach emphasizes the consumption of animal products while eliminating plant-based foods, which can be a significant shift for many individuals. To navigate this transition successfully, it's essential to establish achievable milestones that align with your weight loss aspirations and overall health objectives. Rather than aiming for drastic changes, focus on small, incremental goals that build momentum and foster long-term success.

Begin by defining what weight loss means for you personally. This could involve specific targets, such as shedding a certain number of pounds, or broader objectives like fitting into a preferred clothing size or improving energy levels. By personalizing your goals, you create a more meaningful connection to your journey. Additionally, consider the timeline for these goals. Setting a realistic timeframe, such as aiming to lose one to two pounds per week, can help you maintain motivation without the frustration of unrealistic expectations.

In the context of the carnivore diet, it's crucial to understand how to incorporate this eating style into your daily life without overwhelming yourself. Start with manageable changes, such as committing to a meat-based meal plan for a few days each week. Gradually increase the frequency as you become more comfortable with the diet. This step-wise approach not only makes the transition smoother but also allows you to assess how your body responds to the diet. By listening to your body and adjusting your goals accordingly, you can ensure that your weight loss journey remains sustainable and enjoyable.

Budget considerations also play a significant role in setting realistic goals for the carnivore diet. Quality meat can be expensive, but there are strategies to maintain a budget while still focusing on your weight loss ambitions. For example, consider purchasing in bulk, choosing less expensive cuts of meat, or incorporating organ meats, which offer nutritional benefits at a lower cost. By setting financial parameters alongside your dietary goals, you can create a comprehensive plan that respects both your health aspirations and your budget.

Finally, remember to celebrate small victories along the way. Whether it's reaching a particular weight loss milestone, successfully adapting to a new meal plan, or simply feeling more energetic, recognizing these achievements can boost your motivation. Setting realistic goals is not just about the end result; it's about the journey itself. Embrace the process, adjust your targets as needed, and stay focused on cultivating a sustainable lifestyle that aligns with your carnivore diet journey. By doing so, you'll not only achieve your weight loss goals but also foster a healthier relationship with food and your body.

Preparing Mentally for the Transition

Preparing mentally for the transition to a carnivore diet is a crucial step that often gets overlooked. This journey is not just about changing your food choices but also about altering your mindset and expectations. As you prepare to embrace a meat-based lifestyle, it's essential to acknowledge that this shift may come with challenges that require mental resilience and adaptability. Understanding the psychological aspects of dietary changes can pave the way for a smoother transition and help you maintain your new habits.

First and foremost, it is important to set realistic expectations. The carnivore diet can yield impressive results for weight loss and overall health, but the journey may not be linear. It is common to experience initial fluctuations in weight and energy levels. Some individuals may face cravings for carbohydrates or find it difficult to adjust to a new eating pattern. Remind yourself that it's normal to encounter obstacles during this transition. By setting achievable goals and recognizing that progress may take time, you can foster a mindset geared towards long-term success rather than immediate perfection.

Another vital aspect of mental preparation is educating yourself about the carnivore diet. Familiarize yourself with its principles, nutritional benefits, and potential challenges. Understanding the science behind why a meat-based diet can be effective for weight loss can bolster your confidence and commitment. Knowledge equips you to make informed decisions, whether you're shopping for budget-friendly meats or navigating social situations involving food. Moreover, having a solid grasp of the diet's rationale can help you counter any external skepticism or pressure from friends and family.

Creating a supportive environment is equally important in mental preparation. Surround yourself with individuals who understand or share your dietary goals, whether through online communities, local groups, or friends who are also interested in the carnivore diet. Engaging with others on a similar journey can provide motivation, accountability, and a platform for sharing tips and experiences. Additionally, consider keeping a journal to document your thoughts, feelings, and progress throughout the transition. This practice can serve as a reflective tool to help you understand your motivations and challenges better.

Lastly, be prepared to cultivate patience and resilience. The carnivore diet, while simple in its food choices, can still challenge your old habits and routines. There may be moments of doubt, cravings, or even social situations that test your commitment. By mentally preparing for these scenarios in advance and developing strategies to cope, you can strengthen your resolve. Remind yourself why you chose this diet: to achieve your weight loss goals and improve your overall health. Embracing this mental preparation will not only ease the transition but also enhance your ability to stick to the carnivore lifestyle in the long run.

Chapter 3: Budgeting for Meat

Understanding Meat Prices

The cost of meat is a significant consideration for anyone embracing a carnivore diet, particularly for those on a budget. Prices can vary widely depending on factors such as the type of meat, the cut, the source, and the region. Understanding these variables is essential for making informed purchasing decisions that align with both dietary goals and financial constraints. By familiarizing yourself with the factors that influence meat prices, you can better navigate the marketplace and find strategies to keep your diet affordable.

One of the primary factors affecting meat prices is the type of meat itself. Beef, chicken, pork, and lamb each have different price points based on supply and demand dynamics. For instance, beef tends to be more expensive due to its longer production cycle and higher feed costs. Conversely, chicken is often more budget-friendly, making it a popular choice for those looking to maintain a meat-centric diet without overspending. Understanding these distinctions allows you to prioritize your purchases and consider substitutions that can help keep costs down while still adhering to your dietary preferences.

Cuts of meat also play a crucial role in pricing. Premium cuts like filet mignon or ribeye are often priced at a premium, while tougher cuts, such as chuck roast or brisket, can be much more affordable. These less popular cuts often require longer cooking times but can be incredibly flavorful and satisfying when prepared correctly. Learning to cook with a variety of cuts can not only diversify your meals but also significantly reduce your grocery bills. Exploring local butcher shops or farmer's markets can also yield unexpected bargains on high-quality meat.

Seasonality and local availability are additional factors influencing meat prices. Certain meats may be more expensive during specific times of the year, particularly around holidays or during peak demand seasons. Keeping an eye on sales and seasonal promotions can lead to significant savings. Additionally, sourcing meat from local farms can sometimes offer better prices compared to large grocery chains, especially if you buy in bulk or take advantage of community-supported agriculture (CSA) programs. These strategies can help you build a robust meat supply while minimizing costs.

Lastly, understanding the broader economic factors that impact meat prices, such as feed costs, transportation, and market fluctuations, can provide insight into why prices may rise or fall. Staying informed about these trends can empower you to make proactive decisions about when and where to purchase your meat. By combining this knowledge with practical shopping strategies—such as buying in bulk, freezing excess meat, or taking advantage of sales—you can effectively manage your meat expenses and stay committed to your carnivore diet without sacrificing your budget. Embracing these strategies will not only support your weight loss goals but also enhance your overall experience on the carnivore diet.

Choosing Cost-Effective Cuts of Meat

Choosing cost-effective cuts of meat is essential for anyone embarking on the carnivore diet, especially for beginners who are mindful of their budget. The carnivore diet emphasizes the consumption of animal products while eliminating carbohydrates, making it vital to select cuts of meat that provide nutritional value without straining your finances. By understanding the various cuts of meat available and their associated costs, you can craft a satisfying and healthful diet without overspending.

When shopping for meat, it is crucial to recognize that more expensive cuts do not always equate to better nutrition or flavor. Often, less popular cuts, such as chuck roast, brisket, or pork shoulder, can be just as nutritious and flavorful when prepared correctly. These cuts come from well-exercised muscles, which results in a richer taste and texture. By experimenting with different cooking techniques, such as slow cooking or braising, you can transform these budget-friendly cuts into delicious meals that align with your carnivore lifestyle.

Another effective strategy for saving money on meat is to purchase in bulk. Many local butcher shops and farms offer discounts for buying larger quantities, allowing you to stock up on cuts you enjoy. This approach not only reduces the overall cost per pound but also ensures that you have a steady supply of meat on hand, making it easier to stick to your carnivore diet. Additionally, consider freezing portions for later use, which can help minimize waste and extend the life of your meat supplies.

Incorporating organ meats into your diet is another excellent way to save money while maximizing nutritional benefits. Cuts like liver, heart, and kidneys are often significantly cheaper than traditional muscle meats and are packed with essential vitamins and minerals. For beginners, this may seem daunting, but starting with small amounts and exploring various recipes can help ease the transition. By embracing organ meats, you diversify your diet while keeping costs low, which is particularly beneficial for those focused on weight loss.

Finally, being strategic about your meat purchases can also involve timing and location. Taking advantage of sales, seasonal discounts, or local farmers' markets can lead to substantial savings. Planning your meals around these deals not only helps you stay within budget but also encourages a varied diet, which is important for overall health. By keeping an eye on your local grocery ads and exploring different shopping venues, you can make informed decisions that align with both your dietary goals and financial constraints. Embracing these strategies will empower you to thrive on the carnivore diet without overspending, setting a strong foundation for your weight loss journey.

Seasonal Shopping and Bulk Buying

Seasonal shopping and bulk buying are two essential strategies for those embarking on a carnivore diet, especially when aiming to maintain a budget. By understanding the seasonal availability of various meats and leveraging bulk purchasing options, beginners can significantly cut down on costs while ensuring a diverse and nutritious diet. This approach not only supports weight loss goals but also helps in creating a sustainable eating pattern that aligns with the principles of the carnivore diet.

Seasonal shopping involves purchasing meat and animal products that are at their peak availability during specific times of the year. For instance, certain cuts of beef may be more affordable during the fall when cattle are typically harvested. Similarly, spring might offer better prices on lamb, while summer months could see a surplus of chicken and pork. By planning purchases around these seasonal trends, individuals can take advantage of lower prices and fresher products. Furthermore, seasonal meats often have better flavor profiles and improved quality, making meals more enjoyable without extra costs.

Bulk buying complements the seasonal shopping strategy by allowing individuals to purchase larger quantities of meat at a reduced price per unit. Many grocery stores and butcher shops offer discounts for bulk purchases, which can lead to significant savings over time. For those new to the carnivore diet, this means they can stock up on preferred cuts of meat and freeze them for later use. When buying in bulk, it's crucial to have a plan for proper storage and defrosting, ensuring that the quality of the meat is maintained and waste is minimized. Investing in a good-quality freezer can pay off in the long run, providing a steady supply of meat without the need to frequently shop.

In addition to traditional grocery stores, exploring local farmers' markets and co-ops can uncover further opportunities for seasonal shopping and bulk buying. These venues often sell grass-fed, pasture-raised meats that can be more aligned with the principles of the carnivore diet. Establishing relationships with local farmers can lead to unique bulk buying options, such as purchasing a whole cow or pig, which can be divided among friends or family to further reduce costs. Such collaborative efforts not only promote a sense of community but also ensure that high-quality meats are accessible at budget-friendly prices.

For beginners, transitioning to a carnivore diet can present challenges, particularly when it comes to meal planning and budgeting. Seasonal shopping and bulk buying can ease these challenges by reducing the frequency of shopping trips and offering a clearer path to meal preparation. With a well-stocked freezer, individuals can create a variety of meals without the stress of last-minute grocery runs. This approach also simplifies the budgeting process, as knowing the costs associated with bulk purchases can help in setting realistic financial goals, ultimately supporting weight loss efforts.

In conclusion, seasonal shopping and bulk buying are vital tactics for anyone pursuing a meat-based diet on a budget. By timing purchases according to seasonal fluctuations and taking advantage of bulk discounts, individuals can enjoy a diverse and nutritious carnivore diet without overspending. These strategies not only contribute to achieving weight loss goals but also help form sustainable habits that enhance the overall eating experience. Embracing these methods can empower beginners on their journey, making the carnivore diet both accessible and enjoyable.

Chapter 4: Essential Tools and Equipment

Kitchen Tools for Meat Preparation

In the journey towards embracing the carnivore diet, having the right kitchen tools for meat preparation is essential. These tools not only enhance the cooking experience but also ensure that you can efficiently and effectively prepare nutritious meals without overspending. Whether you are a novice in the kitchen or a seasoned cook, understanding the essential tools and their uses can make a significant difference in your meal preparation process, ultimately supporting your weight loss goals.

First and foremost, a good quality chef's knife is an indispensable tool for any meat preparation. This versatile knife allows for precise cuts, whether you're chopping, slicing, or dicing. Investing in a durable, sharp chef's knife may seem like a splurge, but it pays off in the long run by making meal prep quicker and safer. Additionally, a cutting board is essential for protecting your countertops and maintaining the integrity of your knife. Opt for a sturdy, non-porous cutting board that is easy to clean and won't harbor bacteria, especially when working with raw meat.

Another critical tool in meat preparation is a meat thermometer. Achieving the perfect doneness is crucial not only for flavor but also for food safety. A reliable meat thermometer ensures that your meats are cooked to the appropriate temperatures, which is especially important when following the carnivore diet, where meat is the primary food source. This tool can help prevent overcooking, preserving the juiciness and flavor of your meats while also helping you adhere to your dietary goals.

For those who enjoy marinating or seasoning meats, a set of mixing bowls and measuring spoons can prove invaluable. These tools allow for easy mixing of marinades, rubs, or spices, enabling you to experiment with flavors without straying from your budget. Simple recipes using basic seasonings can elevate the taste of inexpensive cuts of meat, making them more enjoyable and satisfying. Additionally, having a good set of kitchen shears can aid in trimming excess fat and portioning meat, allowing for greater control over the quality of your meals.

Lastly, consider investing in a slow cooker or instant pot. These appliances can transform less expensive cuts of meat into tender, flavorful meals with minimal effort. By utilizing these tools, you can prepare large batches of food, saving both time and money. Cooking in bulk not only helps reduce costs but also simplifies meal planning, which is essential for anyone following the carnivore diet on a budget. With the right kitchen tools, you can streamline your meat preparation process, making it easier to enjoy delicious, satisfying meals that align with your weight loss and dietary goals.

Meal Prep Containers

Meal prep containers are an essential tool for anyone embarking on the carnivore diet, especially for beginners and those looking to maintain this meat-based lifestyle on a budget. These containers not only simplify meal organization but also play a crucial role in portion control and minimizing food waste. By investing in meal prep containers, individuals can streamline their cooking process, allowing for more efficient meal planning and execution. This becomes particularly vital when following a diet that emphasizes high protein and fat intake, as it ensures that meals are ready to grab and go, fitting seamlessly into a busy lifestyle.

When choosing meal prep containers, consider durability and versatility. Opt for options made of glass or high-quality BPA-free plastic that can withstand temperature changes, allowing for both microwave use and freezer storage. Glass containers, while often more expensive, have the advantage of being non-porous and easy to clean, which is beneficial when dealing with fatty meats that can leave residues in cheaper plastic containers. Additionally, having a variety of container sizes will enable you to store different types of meals, from larger portions of proteins to smaller servings of sides or snacks.

Portion control is another significant benefit of using meal prep containers on the carnivore diet. By pre-portioning meals, you can avoid overeating and ensure that you are sticking to your dietary goals. This is particularly important for those focused on weight loss, as it helps in managing caloric intake without the need for constant measuring. Consider investing in containers with compartments, which can help separate different components of your meals, such as meats, fats, and any permissible sides, making it easier to maintain a balanced intake throughout the day.

Meal prep not only saves time but also reduces the temptation to stray from your diet. When healthy, carnivore-friendly meals are readily available, it becomes less likely that you'll reach for convenience foods that could derail your progress. This proactive approach to meal preparation can help mitigate the challenges often faced by beginners, such as cravings or the urge to eat out. By having a stockpile of ready-to-eat meals, you can stay focused on your dietary goals and make consistent progress toward weight loss.

Finally, budgeting is a key concern for anyone on the carnivore diet, and meal prep containers can assist in this area as well. By buying meat in bulk and preparing it in advance, you not only save money but also ensure that you are making the most of your purchases. Utilizing containers to freeze portions of cooked meats allows you to take advantage of sales and bulk buys, minimizing waste and maximizing your budget. In this way, meal prep containers are not just a practical tool; they are a strategic asset in achieving and maintaining your weight loss goals while adhering to the carnivore diet.

Essential Cooking Techniques

Mastering essential cooking techniques is key for anyone embarking on the carnivore diet, especially for beginners who wish to maintain a budget-friendly approach. Understanding these methods not only enhances your culinary skills but also helps you make the most of your meat purchases, reducing waste and maximizing flavor. From basic preparation to advanced cooking skills, these techniques can empower you to create delicious, satisfying meals that align with your dietary goals.

One of the foundational techniques in cooking meat is proper seasoning. While the carnivore diet primarily focuses on animal products, seasoning can elevate the natural flavors of your meats without introducing non-carnivore ingredients. Salt is a staple, helping to enhance the taste and texture of meat. Experimenting with different types of salts—like kosher, sea, or Himalayan—can add subtle variations in flavor. Additionally, incorporating spices such as black pepper or garlic powder can provide depth without deviating from the diet's principles. Understanding how to season effectively can transform even the most budget-friendly cuts of meat into gourmet experiences.

Cooking methods also play a crucial role in achieving the best results from your meat. Techniques such as grilling, roasting, and slow cooking can be particularly effective in bringing out the flavors and tenderness of various cuts. Grilling is a quick method that imparts a smoky flavor, making it ideal for steaks and chops. Roasting, often done in the oven, allows larger cuts to cook evenly while retaining moisture. Slow cooking, on the other hand, is perfect for tougher cuts like brisket or chuck roast, as it breaks down connective tissues, resulting in tender, flavorful dishes. Learning these methods can help you select the right cooking technique for your meat, ensuring that each meal is satisfying and enjoyable.

Another essential technique is mastering the art of meat storage and preparation. Properly handling and storing meat not only prolongs its shelf life but also enhances safety and quality. For those on a budget, buying in bulk and freezing portions for later use can significantly reduce costs. Understanding the best practices for thawing meat, such as overnight in the refrigerator or using cold water, is also crucial to maintain texture and flavor. Additionally, preparing meats ahead of time—such as marinating or pre-cooking—can streamline meal prep during the week, making it easier to stick to your carnivore diet goals.

Finally, understanding how to utilize leftover meats can minimize waste and stretch your budget further. Instead of discarding scraps or uneaten portions, consider repurposing them into new dishes. For example, leftover roast can be shredded and added to a hearty soup or transformed into tacos using carnivore-friendly ingredients. This not only saves money but also encourages creativity in the kitchen, allowing you to enjoy a variety of meals while adhering to the carnivore diet. By mastering these essential cooking techniques, you can ensure that your journey into the carnivore lifestyle is both enjoyable and sustainable, paving the way for long-term weight loss success.

Chapter 5: Meal Planning on a Budget

Creating a Weekly Meal Plan

Creating a weekly meal plan is an essential step for anyone embarking on the carnivore diet, especially for those concerned about budget constraints. A well-structured meal plan not only simplifies grocery shopping but also helps ensure that you stay on track with your dietary goals. For beginners, having a clear outline can minimize the challenges that often accompany dietary changes, allowing for a smoother transition into a meat-based lifestyle. This subchapter will provide practical strategies for crafting a weekly meal plan that aligns with both your weight loss objectives and your budgetary considerations.

Start by assessing your dietary needs and preferences. The carnivore diet primarily consists of animal-based foods, which means that your meal planning will focus heavily on meats, fish, and animal-derived products. Consider the types of meat you enjoy, whether it's beef, pork, chicken, or fish. Additionally, think about incorporating organ meats, which are often more affordable and nutritionally dense. By identifying your preferences, you can create a plan that not only supports your weight loss journey but also makes your meals enjoyable.

Next, set a budget for your weekly grocery shopping. The carnivore diet can be cost-effective if you make strategic choices. Look for sales on meat products, and consider buying in bulk or purchasing cuts that are typically less expensive. For example, chuck roast, ground beef, and chicken thighs can be more economical than premium cuts. Planning your meals around these budget-friendly options can help you maintain a satisfying and varied diet without overspending.

Once you have your preferred meats and budget in mind, outline your weekly meals. A practical approach is to designate specific days for particular proteins. For instance, you might have beef on

Mondays and Wednesdays, pork on Tuesdays, and fish on Thursdays. This not only helps in organizing your shopping list but also allows you to explore different cooking methods and flavors throughout the week. Don't forget to include snacks like beef jerky or hard-boiled eggs, which can keep you satiated between meals and provide additional protein without requiring extensive preparation.

Finally, keep track of your progress and adapt your meal plan as needed. As you transition to a carnivore diet, you may discover which foods fuel your body best and which combinations support your weight loss goals. Regularly reviewing your meal plan can lead to adjustments that enhance your experience. If you find a particular recipe or dish is especially satisfying, consider incorporating it more frequently. This dynamic approach not only helps in maintaining motivation but also ensures that your meal plan remains aligned with your evolving preferences and budget. By committing to a consistent meal planning strategy, you can successfully navigate the carnivore diet while keeping your financial goals in sight.

Incorporating Leftovers

Incorporating leftovers into your meal planning is a savvy strategy that not only reduces food waste but also maximizes your budget while adhering to the carnivore diet. This approach allows you to make the most of the meat you purchase, ensuring you get the best value without compromising your dietary goals. Many beginners may overlook the potential of leftovers, often relegating them to simple reheating. However, with a little creativity, leftovers can become the foundation for a variety of satisfying meals that keep you aligned with your carnivore principles.

One of the most effective ways to utilize leftovers is through batch cooking. Preparing larger portions of meat on designated cooking days means you'll have a ready supply of protein-rich meals throughout the week. For instance, roasting a whole chicken or slow-cooking a large cut of beef can yield several servings. Once the initial meal is enjoyed, the leftover meat can be repurposed in different ways, such as shredding it for salads or soups, or even turning it into meatballs or patties. This not only saves time during busy weekdays but also ensures that you constantly have satisfying options available.

When it comes to storage, proper techniques can help preserve the quality of your leftovers. Invest in airtight containers or vacuum-seal bags to keep meats fresh for longer periods. Labeling these containers with dates will also help you keep track of freshness. It's important to remember that certain meats, like cooked beef or pork, can last in the refrigerator for up to four days, while others, like chicken, can remain good for up to three days. Understanding these time frames will help you utilize your leftovers efficiently, reducing the risk of spoilage and waste.

Creativity plays a significant role in transforming leftovers into new meals. For instance, leftover steak can be sliced thinly and used in a stir-fry, while roasted pork might serve as the base for a hearty breakfast hash. Seasoning and sauces can elevate these dishes, providing variety while staying within the carnivore framework. Additionally, consider using bone broth made from leftover bones as a base for soups or stews, adding depth and nutrition to your meals without extra cost. These techniques not only keep your diet interesting but also reinforce the value of resourcefulness in a meat-centric eating plan.

Lastly, incorporating leftovers into your meal prep routine fosters a sustainable approach to the carnivore diet. By maximizing the use of all parts of the meat you purchase, you not only save money but also contribute to a more environmentally friendly practice by minimizing waste. As you become more accustomed to this method, your confidence in the kitchen will grow, allowing you to experiment more freely with different cuts of meat and preparation styles. Embracing leftovers as a staple of your carnivore journey will ultimately support your weight loss goals while enhancing your overall experience on this fulfilling diet.

Simple Recipes for Beginners

In the journey of adopting a carnivore diet, especially for beginners, simplicity is key. Simple recipes can ease the transition and help newcomers stay on track without feeling overwhelmed. This subchapter presents a selection of straightforward recipes that require minimal ingredients and preparation time, making it easier to embrace a meat-based lifestyle while adhering to a budget. Each recipe is designed to be both accessible and satisfying, allowing you to focus on your weight loss goals without sacrificing flavor or nutrition.

One of the easiest recipes to start with is the classic pan-seared steak. Choose budget-friendly cuts like flank steak or sirloin, which can often be found at a lower price point. Simply season the meat with salt and pepper, then cook it in a hot skillet with a bit of oil. Searing the steak for a few minutes on each side will create a delicious crust, while keeping the inside juicy and tender. This dish not only highlights the natural flavors of the beef, but it also provides a rich source of protein, essential for those looking to lose weight while maintaining muscle mass.

Another beginner-friendly recipe is roasted chicken thighs. Chicken thighs are typically more affordable than chicken breasts and are packed with flavor and fat, making them an excellent choice for a carnivore diet. To prepare, season the thighs with salt, pepper, and any herbs or spices you enjoy. Place them skin-side up on a baking sheet and roast in the oven until crispy and cooked through. This recipe is not only simple but also yields leftovers that can be used for salads or quick meals throughout the week, helping you save both time and money.

For those who enjoy quick meals, scrambled eggs with bacon is a perfect option. Eggs are an excellent source of protein and healthy fats, while bacon adds flavor and satisfaction. Start by cooking the bacon in a skillet until crisp, then remove it and use the rendered fat to scramble the eggs. This recipe can be prepared in under 10 minutes and offers a hearty breakfast that will keep you full and energized. Additionally, eggs are often very affordable, making this dish a budget-friendly choice for anyone on the carnivore diet.

Lastly, consider preparing a simple beef broth. This is a great way to utilize leftover bones from other meals, maximizing your budget while minimizing waste. To make broth, simmer the bones in water with a splash of vinegar for several hours. The result is a nutrient-dense liquid that can be enjoyed on its own or used as a base for soups or sauces. Not only is beef broth rich in collagen and minerals, but it also serves as a comforting and filling option to help curb hunger between meals, supporting your weight loss journey on the carnivore diet.

These simple recipes serve as a foundation for beginners embarking on a carnivore diet on a budget. By focusing on minimal ingredients and straightforward cooking methods, you can create satisfying meals that align with your weight loss goals. As you become more comfortable in the kitchen, feel free to experiment with different cuts of meat and seasonings, tailoring each recipe to your taste while maintaining the core principles of the carnivore diet.

Chapter 6: Overcoming Common Challenges

Dealing with Cravings

Dealing with cravings is a common challenge for anyone embarking on a new dietary journey, especially when transitioning to the carnivore diet. This diet, which primarily consists of animal products, can initially provoke cravings for carbohydrates and other non-meat foods that were staples in your previous eating habits. Understanding the nature of these cravings and developing strategies to manage them is crucial for maintaining adherence to the carnivore diet, particularly for beginners who may find the shift overwhelming.

First, it's essential to recognize that cravings often stem from both physiological and psychological factors. Initially, your body may be adjusting to a sudden decrease in carbohydrates, which can lead to withdrawal-like symptoms. This phase is temporary but can be uncomfortable. To combat this, ensure that you are consuming enough calories from meat, as a lack of energy can exacerbate cravings. Incorporating high-fat cuts of meat can help keep you satiated, making it less likely that you will experience those nagging urges for sugary or starchy foods.

In addition to physical hunger, psychological cravings can be triggered by habits or emotional associations with certain foods. For example, if you are used to snacking on chips while watching television, the urge to indulge in similar snacks can arise even when you are not genuinely hungry. To address this, consider finding alternative routines that do not revolve around food. Engaging in activities such as going for a walk, practicing a hobby, or even starting a new fitness regimen can help distract you from cravings and reinforce your commitment to the carnivore diet.

Meal planning and preparation can also play a significant role in managing cravings. By having a variety of meat-based dishes readily available, you reduce the temptation to reach for non-carnivore options. Batch cooking and storing meals in advance can help prevent last-minute decisions when cravings strike. Additionally, experimenting with different animal products—such as organ meats, fish, and various cuts of beef—can keep your meals interesting and satisfying, which may lessen the desire for foods outside of your diet.

Lastly, patience is key when dealing with cravings. As your body adjusts to the carnivore diet, cravings will likely diminish over time. Staying committed to your goals and reminding yourself of the benefits of this dietary approach can provide motivation. Whether you are seeking weight loss or simply a healthier lifestyle, understanding that cravings are a natural part of the process will help you navigate this journey successfully. With time, the desire for non-carnivore foods will lessen, allowing you to fully embrace the benefits of your new eating habits.

Navigating Social Situations

Navigating social situations while adhering to the carnivore diet can be a daunting challenge, particularly for beginners. Social gatherings often revolve around food, and traditional meal options may not align with a meat-centric lifestyle. To successfully navigate these scenarios, it is essential to approach them with a proactive mindset. Planning ahead, communicating your dietary preferences, and finding creative ways to participate in social events can make the experience more enjoyable and less stressful.

One effective strategy is to prepare in advance for social gatherings. Consider bringing your own dish that aligns with the carnivore diet. This not only ensures you have something to eat that meets your dietary needs but also provides an opportunity to share your culinary skills with others. A simple yet delicious option could be a meat platter featuring a variety of cooked meats, such as grilled steak, roasted chicken, or even homemade meatballs. By contributing to the meal, you can avoid potential social awkwardness and demonstrate that eating carnivorously can be both satisfying and appealing.

Communication is key when it comes to social situations. Inform friends and family about your dietary choices ahead of time, which allows them to accommodate your needs. This approach fosters understanding and can lead to more inclusive gatherings where everyone feels comfortable. If you're attending a potluck or a restaurant, don't hesitate to express your preferences or ask about available options. Most people appreciate transparency, and you may even inspire them to learn more about the carnivore diet, sparking interesting conversations.

Flexibility plays a crucial role in successfully navigating social situations. While it's important to stick to your dietary goals, being too rigid can lead to feelings of isolation or frustration. If a particular event presents limited options, consider making compromises that still align closely with your dietary principles. For instance, if all that's available is a meat-based dish with non-carnivore sides, focus on enjoying the protein while minimizing the non-compliant items. This way, you can participate in the social aspect without feeling deprived or guilty about straying from your diet.

Lastly, remember that social situations are about connection and enjoyment, not just food. Engage in conversations, participate in activities, and focus on the company around you rather than solely on the meal. By prioritizing relationships and experiences, you can successfully navigate social gatherings while maintaining your commitment to the carnivore diet. Embracing a positive outlook and employing these strategies will not only help you stick to your dietary goals but also enhance your social life as you embark on this new and exciting journey.

Managing Energy Levels

Managing energy levels is crucial for anyone embarking on the carnivore diet, especially for beginners seeking to lose weight while adhering to a meat-based regimen. The transition to a diet primarily composed of animal products can result in fluctuations in energy, as the body adapts to a new source of fuel. Understanding how to effectively manage these energy levels can enhance overall well-being, improve exercise performance, and support weight loss goals.

One of the first steps in managing energy levels on a carnivore diet is to establish a consistent eating schedule. Regular meal timing can help stabilize blood sugar levels and prevent energy crashes that often accompany drastic dietary changes. For beginners, it may be beneficial to start with three meals a day, focusing on nutrient-dense cuts of meat that provide ample protein and fat. Incorporating organ meats can also boost nutrient intake, promoting sustained energy throughout the day. As individuals become more accustomed to the diet, they can experiment with meal frequency to find what works best for their energy needs.

Hydration plays a vital role in energy management, particularly when transitioning to a carnivore diet. Many beginners may overlook the importance of adequate water intake, especially since animal-based diets can be lower in carbohydrates, which typically contribute to water retention. It's essential to drink enough water daily to support metabolic processes and maintain optimal energy levels. Additionally, incorporating electrolytes can help prevent fatigue and maintain hydration, especially if the body is shedding excess water weight during the initial stages of the diet.

Sleep quality is another critical factor in energy management. The carnivore diet can initially disrupt sleep patterns for some individuals due to changes in nutrient intake and hormonal adjustments. Prioritizing sleep hygiene—such as maintaining a regular sleep schedule, creating a comfortable sleep environment, and minimizing screen time before bed—can significantly impact energy levels during the day. A well-rested body is more resilient and better equipped to handle the challenges of dietary changes, making it easier to stay on track with weight loss goals.

Lastly, incorporating physical activity into a daily routine can help regulate energy levels while promoting weight loss. Beginners should aim to find an exercise regimen that complements their lifestyle and energy capacity. Low-impact activities, such as walking or light resistance training, can be particularly beneficial during the initial transition period. As energy levels stabilize, individuals may feel inclined to increase the intensity and frequency of their workouts. By listening to their bodies and adjusting activity levels accordingly, individuals can harness the benefits of exercise to enhance energy management and support their overall weight loss journey on the carnivore diet.

Chapter 7: Transitioning to the Carnivore Diet

Phased Approach to Transition

The transition to the carnivore diet can be both exciting and daunting, especially for those accustomed to a more varied diet. A phased approach to this transition allows individuals to acclimate gradually, minimizing potential discomfort and making the process more manageable. This method not only eases the body into a new way of eating but also provides an opportunity to identify and address any challenges that may arise along the way. By breaking the transition into distinct phases, individuals can set realistic goals, monitor their progress, and adapt their strategies as needed.

The first phase of the transition involves a gradual reduction of non-carnivorous foods. This step is crucial for those who may have relied heavily on carbohydrates or processed foods. Begin by eliminating one food group at a time, starting with grains and sugars, which can lead to cravings and withdrawal symptoms. For example, spend a week focusing on reducing your intake of bread, pasta, and sweets. This allows your body to adjust without overwhelming it. During this phase, it's essential to increase your intake of meat and animal products gradually, ensuring that your body starts to adapt to the new macronutrient profile.

Once the initial transition is underway, the second phase introduces a more structured carnivore eating plan. At this point, individuals should focus on incorporating a variety of meats, including beef, pork, poultry, and fish, as well as animal-based products like eggs and dairy. Experimenting with different cuts and cooking methods can make this phase enjoyable and prevent monotony. Setting a budget is critical here; by prioritizing cheaper cuts of meat, such as ground beef or chicken thighs, you can maintain a carnivore diet without overspending. Utilizing sales and bulk buying can further enhance your budget strategy while ensuring you have a steady supply of protein-rich foods.

The third phase is about fine-tuning your carnivore diet to suit your personal preferences and nutritional needs. This may involve tracking your food intake to understand how different meats and animal products affect your energy levels, digestion, and overall well-being. Some individuals may find that they thrive on a specific ratio of fatty to lean meats, while others may require more organ meats for optimal health. This phase encourages self-exploration and customization, allowing each person to create a diet that works best for them, all while keeping a close eye on costs through careful planning.

Finally, the fourth phase focuses on maintaining the carnivore diet in the long term. This phase is essential for ensuring that the transition sticks and that you do not revert to previous eating habits. Establishing a routine around meal planning, shopping, and cooking can help solidify this new lifestyle. Consider joining support groups or online communities where you can share experiences and gain insights from others on a similar journey. Keeping track of your progress, celebrating milestones, and adjusting your budget and meal plans as necessary will not only help in sustaining a meat-based diet but also contribute to ongoing weight loss and health improvements.

In summary, a phased approach to transitioning to the carnivore diet allows beginners to adapt at a comfortable pace while addressing potential challenges. By systematically reducing non-carnivorous foods, introducing a variety of meats, fine-tuning the diet to personal needs, and establishing long-term maintenance strategies, individuals can successfully embark on their journey toward a healthier, meat-based lifestyle without breaking the bank. This methodical strategy not only supports weight loss but also encourages a sustainable approach to the carnivore diet, making it accessible for everyone.

Detox Symptoms and How to Handle Them

Detox symptoms can arise during the initial phase of transitioning to a carnivore diet, particularly for those who are accustomed to a higher intake of carbohydrates and processed foods. As the body adjusts to a new source of energy, it may go through a period of discomfort. This phase, often referred to as the "keto flu" or simply detox symptoms, can manifest as headaches, fatigue, irritability, digestive changes, and even cravings for sugar and carbs. Understanding these symptoms is crucial for anyone embarking on this meat-based journey, as it can help demystify the experience and provide strategies for coping.

One common symptom of detoxification is fatigue. This occurs as the body shifts from using glucose as its primary energy source to relying on fat. While this adjustment can be challenging, increasing hydration can alleviate some of the fatigue. Drinking plenty of water, perhaps infused with electrolytes, can help maintain energy levels and reduce feelings of lethargy. Additionally, ensuring that you're getting adequate salt can support electrolyte balance and help combat fatigue during this transitional period.

Headaches are another prevalent symptom experienced by many newcomers to the carnivore diet. This discomfort is often linked to withdrawal from sugar and carbohydrates, which the body may be accustomed to relying on for quick energy. To manage headaches, consider implementing gradual changes to your diet rather than an abrupt shift. This might involve slowly reducing carbohydrate intake over several days before fully committing to the carnivore diet. Moreover, regular meals rich in fatty cuts of meat can help stabilize blood sugar levels, potentially reducing the frequency and intensity of headaches.

Digestive changes are also common as your body adjusts to a diet composed primarily of animal products. These changes can include constipation or diarrhea, which may be unsettling for beginners. To navigate these symptoms effectively, focus on incorporating a variety of meat types into your diet, including organ meats and fatty cuts, which can provide essential nutrients and promote digestive health. Additionally, gradually introducing more animal-based foods rather than overwhelming your system with a sudden influx of protein can help ease digestive discomfort.

Lastly, cravings for sugar and carbohydrates can be a significant challenge during the detox phase. These cravings are typically a result of the body's reliance on glucose and can be particularly strong in the first few days. To combat these urges, keep your meals satisfying and nutrient-dense, focusing on high-fat cuts of meat that can help curb hunger and provide lasting energy. Engaging in activities that distract you from cravings, such as exercise or hobbies, can also be beneficial. Over time, as your body adapts to the carnivore diet, these cravings will likely diminish, paving the way for a more sustainable approach to weight loss and overall health.

Monitoring Your Body's Response

Monitoring your body's response is an essential aspect of embarking on the carnivore diet journey, especially for beginners focused on weight loss. As you transition to a meat-based diet, it is crucial to pay attention to how your body reacts to the significant dietary shift. This includes observing changes in energy levels, digestion, mood, and overall well-being. Keeping a journal can be an effective way to track these changes, allowing you to identify patterns and adjust your approach as needed. By understanding your body's cues, you can optimize your diet for better results and ensure you are on the right path toward your weight loss goals.

One of the first indicators to monitor is your energy levels. Many individuals experience a period of adjustment when switching to the carnivore diet, which can include fatigue or low energy as your body adapts to burning fat for fuel instead of carbohydrates. It is important to note that this phase is temporary for most people. Keeping track of your energy fluctuations throughout the day can help you identify when you feel most energized and when you might need to adjust your meal timing or composition. Additionally, paying attention to your sleep patterns can provide insights into how well your diet supports restful nights and rejuvenating mornings.

Digestion is another critical area to observe as you navigate the carnivore diet. Some individuals may experience changes in bowel movements or digestive discomfort during the initial transition. This can be due to the increased intake of protein and fat compared to a carbohydrate-heavy diet. Monitoring your digestive health will help you determine which types of meats work best for your body. For instance, fatty cuts of meat may be more satisfying and easier on the stomach for some, while others may prefer leaner options. Keeping a food diary that includes how you feel after each meal can be beneficial in pinpointing what works for you.

Moreover, emotional and mental well-being can also be influenced by dietary changes. Many people report improvements in mood and mental clarity when adopting a carnivore diet, but it is essential to assess your own experiences. Changes in mood, anxiety levels, and cognitive function can all be impacted by dietary shifts. Tracking these emotional responses alongside your physical changes will provide a more comprehensive view of how the carnivore diet is affecting you. If you notice negative changes, consider consulting with a healthcare professional or nutritionist to help you navigate these challenges.

Finally, it is important to remain patient and flexible during this monitoring phase. The carnivore diet may not yield immediate results, and everyone's experience is unique. Regularly evaluating your body's response allows for informed adjustments to your meal plans and lifestyle. Remember, the goal is to find a sustainable approach that fits your individual needs and supports your weight loss journey. By staying attuned to your body and making necessary changes, you can successfully navigate the carnivore diet while maintaining your budget and achieving your health goals.

Chapter 8: Maintaining Your Carnivore Lifestyle

Sustainable Practices for Long-Term Success

Sustainable practices are essential for anyone embarking on the carnivore diet, especially for individuals focused on weight loss and maintaining a budget. To ensure long-term success, it's important to adopt strategies that not only support health but also make the diet economically feasible. Understanding how to source high-quality meats, manage food waste, and incorporate seasonal eating can lead to a sustainable lifestyle that complements the carnivore approach. This entails a combination of smart purchasing decisions and mindful consumption, ultimately promoting both health and financial savings.

One of the primary ways to maintain a budget-friendly carnivore diet is to prioritize the purchase of whole animals or larger cuts of meat. Buying in bulk can significantly reduce costs per pound, making it easier to stick to a meat-based diet without overspending. Local butcher shops or farmers' markets often offer better deals than large grocery chains. Additionally, exploring community-supported agriculture (CSA) programs that feature meat can provide access to fresh, local products at a lower price. By forging relationships with local suppliers, individuals can gain valuable insights into seasonal availability and potentially secure discounts for bulk purchases, enhancing both sustainability and savings.

Incorporating seasonal eating into the carnivore diet is another sustainable practice that aligns with both health and budget goals. By consuming meats that are in season or locally available, individuals not only support their local economy but also benefit from fresher, more nutrient-dense food. Seasonality can affect meat quality and pricing, making it advantageous to stay informed about what is available throughout the year. Planning meals around these seasonal offerings can lead to more diverse and satisfying dietary choices while keeping costs manageable.

Food waste is a critical issue in any dietary plan, and the carnivore diet is no exception. Developing a habit of using leftover meats, bones, and even organ meats can significantly enhance sustainability. For example, bone broth made from leftover bones is not only nutritious but also a cost-effective way to utilize every part of the animal. Additionally, incorporating organ meats into the diet can provide a wealth of nutrients at a fraction of the cost of muscle meats. By being resourceful and creative in the kitchen, individuals can minimize waste and maximize nutritional intake, ensuring that they make the most of their meat purchases.

Finally, fostering a community around the carnivore diet can serve as an invaluable resource for sustainable practices. Engaging with others who share similar dietary goals can provide support, motivation, and practical tips on budgeting, meal planning, and sourcing ingredients. Online forums, social media groups, and local meetups can facilitate knowledge sharing and help newcomers navigate the challenges of transitioning to a carnivore lifestyle. By building a network of like-minded individuals, it becomes easier to stay committed to the diet while exploring innovative ways to maintain sustainability and achieve long-term success.

Adapting to Changing Circumstances

Adapting to changing circumstances is an essential skill for anyone embarking on a new dietary journey, especially for those exploring the carnivore diet on a budget. The world around us is constantly evolving, and so too are our personal situations, which can impact our ability to stick to a specific eating plan. Whether it's fluctuating food prices, unexpected life events, or shifts in personal health, being able to navigate these changes effectively is crucial for long-term success. This subchapter will provide practical strategies to help you remain committed to your carnivore diet despite the inevitable ups and downs of life.

One of the first steps in adapting to changing circumstances is to stay informed about the market trends related to meat prices.

Understanding seasonal fluctuations can help you plan your grocery shopping more effectively. For instance, certain cuts of meat may be more affordable during specific times of the year, such as summer grilling season or during holiday sales. Regularly checking local flyers, using apps that track grocery prices, and even connecting with local farmers or butcher shops can offer insights into when to buy certain items at the best prices. This proactive approach will not only help you save money but also ensure that you have the necessary resources to maintain your diet.

Another key aspect of adapting is flexibility in your meal planning. While the carnivore diet emphasizes a meat-centric approach, there are various ways to incorporate different types of meats and animal products without straying from your budget. If beef prices rise, consider exploring more economical options like chicken, pork, or even organ meats, which are often overlooked but nutrient-dense and budget-friendly. Additionally, diversifying your protein sources can prevent monotony in your meals, making it easier to sustain your diet in the long run. Keeping a list of versatile recipes that cater to various meats will help you quickly pivot when prices change or when certain meats are unavailable.

Transitioning to the carnivore diet can pose challenges, particularly for beginners who may be accustomed to a more varied diet. If you find yourself facing obstacles such as cravings for non-meat foods or difficulties in meal preparation, it's essential to recognize these challenges as part of the process. Developing a toolkit of coping strategies can aid in overcoming these hurdles. For instance, experimenting with different cooking methods, seasoning techniques, or even meat-based snacks can make the transition smoother. Additionally, seeking support from online communities or local groups can provide encouragement and tips from those who have successfully navigated similar challenges.

Lastly, maintaining a positive mindset during times of change is vital for achieving your weight loss goals on the carnivore diet. Embrace the idea that setbacks are a natural part of any journey, and cultivating resilience will empower you to adapt without losing sight of your objectives. Keeping a journal to record your experiences, feelings, and progress can serve as a powerful tool for reflection and motivation. By focusing on your achievements, no matter how small, you reinforce your commitment to your goals and create a mental framework that encourages perseverance.

In conclusion, adapting to changing circumstances on the carnivore diet requires a blend of practical strategies and a resilient mindset. By staying informed about market trends, being flexible in your meal planning, developing coping strategies for challenges, and maintaining a positive outlook, you can navigate the complexities of this dietary lifestyle without compromising your budget or goals. As you continue on this journey, remember that adaptability is not just about surviving change; it's about thriving in the face of it.

Celebrating Milestones and Progress

Celebrating milestones and progress is an essential aspect of any weight loss journey, particularly when embarking on a specific dietary path such as the carnivore diet. The carnivore diet, which emphasizes the consumption of animal-based foods while eliminating plant-based options, can present unique challenges for beginners. However, recognizing and celebrating each achievement along the way not only boosts motivation but also reinforces the positive changes being made. Whether it's shedding those first few pounds, successfully navigating a budget-friendly shopping trip, or mastering meal prep, acknowledging these milestones helps create a sense of accomplishment and encourages continued dedication.

One of the most significant milestones on the carnivore diet is the initial weight loss. For many beginners, the first few weeks can be transformative, as the body adjusts to a new way of eating. Tracking weight loss progress can be done in various ways—through regular weigh-ins, taking measurements, or noting how clothes fit. Each time you notice a change, whether it's a few pounds lost or a belt loop adjusted, take a moment to appreciate the hard work that led to that result. Additionally, consider sharing your progress with a supportive community. Online forums and social media groups can provide encouragement, tips, and a sense of camaraderie, making the journey feel less isolating.

Another important aspect of celebrating progress lies in mastering the budget-friendly strategies that are integral to the carnivore diet. Shopping for meat on a budget can be daunting, especially for those new to this eating style. Successfully finding ways to save money—like buying in bulk, choosing less expensive cuts, or utilizing local resources such as farmers' markets—deserves recognition. Each time you successfully stick to your budget while still enjoying delicious, nourishing meals, it reinforces the idea that living this lifestyle is not only achievable but sustainable. Documenting these strategies and sharing them with others can foster a sense of community and inspire newcomers to pursue their carnivore journey without the financial strain.

Transitioning to the carnivore diet can also bring about a range of physical and mental milestones. Many individuals report increased energy levels, improved mental clarity, and reduced cravings as they adapt to this new way of eating. Celebrating these non-scale victories is just as important as tracking weight loss. Keeping a journal to note changes in energy, mood, or overall well-being can serve as a powerful reminder of why you began this journey. Reflecting on these improvements can boost your motivation, especially during challenging moments when you might feel tempted to revert to old habits.

Lastly, as you reach key milestones, it's crucial to set new goals to continue your journey. Whether it's trying a new meat-based recipe, experimenting with different cooking techniques, or exploring new sources of protein, setting these objectives can keep your experience fresh and engaging. Each new challenge you undertake not only expands your culinary repertoire but also reinforces your commitment to the carnivore lifestyle. Celebrating these ongoing achievements—no matter how small—creates a positive feedback loop that keeps you moving forward, ultimately leading to lasting success in your weight loss journey on the carnivore diet.

-

-

-

-

Chapter 9: Success Stories and Testimonials

Real-Life Transformations

Real-life transformations serve as powerful motivators for anyone considering the carnivore diet, particularly those seeking effective weight loss strategies without overspending. In this subchapter, we will explore various success stories that demonstrate how individuals have embraced this meat-based lifestyle, shedding pounds while adhering to a budget. These examples will provide insight into the practical application of the carnivore diet and the potential benefits it offers for beginners.

One of the most compelling aspects of the carnivore diet is its simplicity. Many newcomers find that by focusing solely on animal products, they can streamline their meal planning and shopping. Take the story of Sarah, a busy mother of three who struggled with weight gain after pregnancy. By switching to a carnivore diet, she discovered that her grocery bills actually decreased. By purchasing bulk meats and prioritizing cost-effective options like ground beef and chicken thighs, Sarah not only lost over 30 pounds in six months but also simplified her dinner routine, allowing her more time to spend with her family.

In addition to weight loss, real-life transformations often highlight the health benefits associated with the carnivore diet. For instance, Tom, a 45-year-old office worker, experienced significant improvements in his energy levels and mental clarity after committing to a meat-based regimen. Initially skeptical about the diet's effects, Tom was pleasantly surprised to find that his cravings for processed foods diminished over time. He focused on affordable cuts of meat, utilizing sales and local butcher shops to stay within budget. Tom's journey illustrates that the carnivore diet can lead not only to weight loss but also to enhanced overall well-being, making it an appealing choice for beginners.

Transitioning to a carnivore diet can present challenges, but many individuals find innovative solutions to overcome them. For example, Lisa, a college student, initially faced financial constraints when starting her carnivore journey. By prioritizing seasonal meats and exploring local farmer's markets, she learned to navigate her limited budget effectively. Lisa's resourcefulness allowed her to maintain a balanced diet while enjoying a variety of flavors and textures. Her experience underscores the importance of adaptability and creativity when adopting a new eating style, especially for those concerned about costs.

Finally, the stories of those who have successfully transformed their lives through the carnivore diet highlight the community aspect of this lifestyle. Online forums, social media groups, and local meet-ups provide support, inspiration, and practical tips for beginners. As individuals share their journeys, they reinforce the idea that the carnivore diet is not just a solitary endeavor but a collective movement toward better health and wellness. By learning from others' experiences, newcomers can find the encouragement they need to embark on their own transformations, making the carnivore diet an accessible and empowering choice for weight loss and overall health.

Lessons Learned from Others

Embarking on a carnivore diet can be both exciting and daunting for beginners, especially when trying to maintain a meat-based regimen without overspending. Learning from the experiences of others can provide valuable insights and help navigate potential pitfalls. By examining the strategies, successes, and challenges faced by those who have walked this path before, newcomers can better prepare themselves for their own journey toward weight loss and improved health.

One of the most important lessons gleaned from others is the significance of meal planning and preparation. Many successful practitioners of the carnivore diet emphasize the need to plan meals in advance to avoid impulse purchases and food waste. By creating a weekly menu and shopping list, you can focus on high-quality meats that fit your budget. This proactive approach not only saves money but also ensures that you stay on track with your dietary goals, reducing the temptation to stray from the diet when hunger strikes.

Another key takeaway is the importance of finding local resources for quality meat. Many individuals have discovered that local farmers, butcher shops, and community-supported agriculture (CSA) programs often offer more affordable options compared to larger grocery chains. Building relationships with local suppliers not only supports the community but may also provide access to bulk purchasing discounts or seasonal sales. Engaging with others in the carnivore community can also lead to shared tips and resources for sourcing meat affordably.

Moreover, understanding the value of variety within the carnivore diet can help prevent boredom and enhance the overall experience. Many successful dieters share that incorporating different cuts of meat, organ meats, and various cooking methods can make meals more enjoyable while ensuring a well-rounded nutrient intake. Experimenting with different flavors and textures keeps the diet interesting and can lead to lasting satisfaction, making it easier to adhere to the dietary changes over time.

Lastly, learning from the challenges faced by others can provide crucial insights into effective transitioning strategies. Many beginners encounter difficulties such as cravings, energy fluctuations, or social pressures. Those who have successfully navigated these obstacles often recommend gradual changes, such as slowly reducing carbohydrate intake before fully committing to the diet. Additionally, joining online communities or local support groups can foster a sense of accountability and encouragement, helping to overcome hurdles together. By understanding the experiences of others, newcomers can better equip themselves to face and conquer their own challenges on the carnivore diet journey.

Building a Support Network

Building a support network is a crucial step in successfully adopting the carnivore diet, especially for beginners and those aiming to lose weight on a budget. A well-structured support network can provide motivation, accountability, and valuable information to help navigate the challenges that come with this unique dietary approach. By connecting with others who share similar goals or experiences, you can enhance your journey and make the transition smoother.

Start by identifying the people in your life who can be part of your support network. This may include family members, friends, or colleagues who are open to understanding your dietary choices. Engaging them in conversation about the carnivore diet can foster a supportive environment. Share your goals, the reasons behind your dietary shift, and the benefits you hope to achieve. This openness can encourage them to join you on your journey or at least provide the encouragement you need to stick to your plan.

Online communities play a significant role in building a support network, particularly for those following niche diets like the carnivore diet. Utilize social media platforms, forums, and dedicated websites to connect with like-minded individuals. These spaces often offer valuable resources such as meal ideas, budget-friendly shopping tips, and personal success stories. Participating in discussions and sharing your experiences can help you feel less isolated and more empowered in your dietary choices.

Consider joining local or virtual meetups focused on the carnivore diet. These gatherings can provide opportunities for networking and learning from others who have successfully navigated similar challenges. Many communities have groups that meet regularly to discuss meal planning, budget strategies, and share recipes. Engaging in these interactions can also introduce you to potential workout partners or accountability buddies, reinforcing your commitment to both the diet and your weight loss goals.

Lastly, don't underestimate the power of professional support. If you have access to healthcare providers, nutritionists, or dietitians who understand the carnivore diet, they can offer tailored advice and guidance. They can help you navigate any nutritional concerns and ensure you are meeting your dietary needs without overspending. Whether through one-on-one consultations or group workshops, professional support can be an invaluable resource as you work towards your weight loss objectives on a budget. Building a strong support network empowers you to embrace the carnivore diet confidently, making your journey not only more achievable but also more enjoyable.

Chapter 10: Resources and Further Reading

Recommended Books and Guides

In exploring the Carnivore Diet, newcomers will find a wealth of resources that can guide them on their journey. Recommended books and guides serve as essential tools for understanding the principles behind this meat-based lifestyle and how to adopt it effectively, especially on a budget. These resources not only provide foundational knowledge but also offer practical strategies for overcoming common challenges faced by beginners. By leveraging these readings, individuals can enhance their comprehension of the diet while navigating their journey towards weight loss and overall health.

One highly regarded book for those new to the Carnivore Diet is "The Carnivore Diet" by Dr. Shawn Baker. This comprehensive guide outlines the science behind the diet, explaining how an all-meat regimen can lead to weight loss and improved health outcomes. Dr. Baker shares personal anecdotes and testimonials from those who have successfully transformed their lives through this dietary approach. Additionally, he addresses common misconceptions and pitfalls, providing readers with the confidence to embrace the lifestyle while on a budget. This book serves as both an introduction and a motivational tool for beginners.

Another valuable resource is "Meat: A Love Story" by Susannah Smith.

This book takes a unique approach by combining personal narrative with practical advice. Smith details her journey into the world of meat-based eating, highlighting the joys and challenges she faced along the way. Her insights into sourcing affordable, high-quality meat make it an excellent guide for those looking to maintain a carnivore diet without straining their finances. Readers can glean tips on shopping smart, meal planning, and making the most of each cut of meat, all of which are critical skills for anyone embarking on this dietary adventure.

For individuals looking for a more structured approach, "The Carnivore Cookbook" by Jessica Haggard offers a plethora of recipes designed specifically for those following a carnivore diet. This guide not only emphasizes the importance of simplicity in meal preparation but also showcases how to create satisfying and enjoyable dishes while adhering to budget constraints. Haggard's recipes are accessible and adaptable, making it easier for beginners to incorporate the carnivore diet into their daily lives. The inclusion of budget-friendly meal plans allows readers to visualize how they can sustain this lifestyle without overspending.

Lastly, "Carnivore Cure" by James L. Wilson provides a deeper dive into the health benefits associated with a meat-based diet. Wilson discusses the physiological impacts of eliminating carbohydrates and how this shift can lead to significant weight loss and improved well-being. His approach combines scientific research with actionable advice, making it an ideal resource for those who want to understand the "why" behind the diet while implementing it effectively. By engaging with this literature, beginners can arm themselves with knowledge and strategies that foster a successful transition to the Carnivore Diet, ensuring they meet their weight loss goals while staying within their budget.

Online Communities and Forums

Online communities and forums have emerged as invaluable resources for those embarking on the carnivore diet, particularly for beginners and those looking to manage their diet on a budget. These platforms offer a space where individuals can share their experiences, ask questions, and find support from others who are navigating the same dietary path. With the rise of social media and specialized websites, it has never been easier to connect with like-minded individuals who are enthusiastic about the benefits of a meat-based diet. This subchapter explores how these online communities can aid in weight loss and provide practical strategies for maintaining the carnivore diet without financial strain.

One of the primary advantages of online communities is the wealth of information they provide. Beginners can access a plethora of tips and strategies shared by seasoned carnivores, which can significantly ease the transition into a meat-based lifestyle. Members often discuss their favorite budget-friendly cuts of meat, where to find deals, and how to maximize the nutritional value of their meals without overspending. These discussions can help newcomers feel more confident in their choices, making it easier to stick with the diet and achieve their weight loss goals.

Support is another critical aspect of these online forums. Weight loss journeys can be challenging, and having a network of individuals who understand the struggles can be incredibly motivating. Whether it's celebrating a milestone or seeking advice during a difficult week, community members offer encouragement and accountability. Many forums have dedicated threads for sharing progress, which can foster a sense of camaraderie and inspire others to persevere in their dietary changes. This emotional support can be just as vital as the practical advice shared, creating an environment conducive to long-term success.

In addition to emotional support, online communities often feature discussions about common challenges faced by those on the carnivore diet. For instance, participants may share their experiences with cravings, meal planning, or the social dynamics that come into play when adhering to a restrictive diet. By openly discussing these challenges, members can develop strategies to overcome them, ensuring that they remain committed to their weight loss goals. Newcomers can learn from the mistakes and triumphs of others, allowing them to navigate potential pitfalls with greater ease.

Finally, online communities can serve as a springboard for learning about new recipes, cooking techniques, and meal prep ideas that fit within a budget. Many members are eager to share their culinary creations, including simple, cost-effective recipes that make the carnivore diet accessible to all. This sharing of knowledge not only helps others save money but also encourages creativity in the kitchen. By participating in these discussions, beginners can expand their culinary repertoire while keeping their grocery bills in check, making the carnivore diet a sustainable choice for weight loss.

Tools and Apps for Tracking Progress

Tracking progress is a crucial component for anyone embarking on a weight loss journey, particularly for beginners adapting to the carnivore diet. As individuals shift from a more traditional diet to one focused solely on animal products, utilizing the right tools and apps can significantly enhance motivation and accountability. These resources not only help you monitor your food intake but also allow you to visualize your progress over time, making adjustments easier and more informed.

One of the most effective tools for tracking progress is a food diary or journal, where you can log your daily meals, snacks, and any other food items consumed. While traditional pen-and-paper methods are effective, digital options have gained popularity due to their convenience and additional features. Apps like MyFitnessPal or Cronometer enable users to enter their food intake and automatically calculate nutritional information. These platforms can be particularly beneficial for carnivore dieters, as they provide insights into macronutrients and micronutrients that are vital for health, ensuring that you're not just focusing on calories but also on the quality of your food.

In addition to food tracking apps, progress tracking tools can include weight and measurement logs. Many users find it motivating to see their weight loss journey represented visually through graphs and charts. Apps like Happy Scale or Libra allow you to input your weight regularly and track trends over time, rather than focusing solely on daily fluctuations. This is particularly important on the carnivore diet, where initial weight loss may be rapid due to water weight, followed by a more gradual decline. Understanding these trends can help maintain motivation and avoid discouragement during plateaus.

For those who enjoy a more holistic approach, combining food tracking with fitness apps can provide a comprehensive view of overall health and wellness. Apps like Fitbit or Apple Health can track physical activity, sleep patterns, and heart rate, which are all essential components of a successful weight loss strategy. By integrating these functionalities, you can correlate your dietary choices with your physical activity, allowing for a better understanding of how your carnivore diet impacts your overall health and fitness goals.

Lastly, it is essential to remember that while technology can be incredibly helpful, it should not become a source of stress or obsession. The goal of tracking progress is to inform and support your journey, not to create anxiety around food choices or weight numbers. Consider setting realistic goals and using these tools as a means of encouragement rather than a strict guideline. This balanced approach will help you stay committed to your carnivore diet while remaining adaptable, ensuring that you can enjoy the journey of weight loss and improved health without breaking the bank.

Chapter 11: Conclusion

Recap of Key Takeaways

In the journey toward embracing the carnivore diet, understanding the key takeaways is essential for both beginners and those looking to maintain a meat-based eating plan without straining their finances. This subchapter offers a recap of the most important concepts discussed throughout the book, providing a succinct overview of strategies to help you navigate the carnivore lifestyle effectively. By focusing on these critical points, readers can reinforce their knowledge and feel more confident about their dietary choices.

One of the central themes of the book is the importance of planning and budgeting. Implementing a carnivore diet does not have to be an expensive endeavor. By learning to shop strategically—such as buying in bulk, choosing less expensive cuts of meat, and utilizing sales and discounts—readers can significantly reduce costs. Emphasizing the need to prioritize quality meat while also being budget-conscious allows newcomers to experience the benefits of the carnivore diet without feeling financial strain.

Additionally, transitioning to a carnivore diet can present challenges, especially for beginners accustomed to a more varied food intake. The book highlights the importance of gradually eliminating non-carnivore foods, which can help mitigate symptoms of withdrawal and digestive discomfort. Understanding the body's adaptation process is crucial; readers are encouraged to listen to their bodies and adjust their diet according to personal responses. This approach fosters a sustainable transition, making it easier to stick with the diet long-term.

Community support also plays a vital role in successfully adopting the carnivore diet. Engaging with online groups or local meetups can provide motivation, accountability, and a wealth of shared knowledge. The book stresses the benefits of connecting with others who are on similar journeys, as this can help beginners overcome common hurdles and learn from the experiences of seasoned practitioners. Building a network of support not only enhances the experience but also encourages adherence to the diet.

Lastly, the overarching message of "Meat Your Goals" is the emphasis on individualization. Each person's journey on the carnivore diet will differ based on their unique health goals, preferences, and budget considerations. The key takeaways encourage readers to experiment and find what works best for them, fostering a personalized approach to nutrition. By focusing on these fundamental principles, individuals can confidently embark on their carnivore diet journey, achieving their weight loss goals while enjoying delicious and satisfying meals.

Encouragement for Your Journey

Embarking on a new diet can be both exciting and daunting, especially when transitioning to a meat-based diet like the carnivore diet. This subchapter serves as a source of encouragement for those who are taking their first steps toward this lifestyle. Understanding that weight loss is a journey filled with ups and downs is crucial. It's essential to remind yourself that progress may not always be linear, but with commitment and the right strategies, you can achieve your goals while adhering to a budget.

One of the key aspects of the carnivore diet is its simplicity, which can be a tremendous advantage for beginners. Unlike other diets that often require counting calories or tracking macronutrients, the carnivore diet focuses primarily on animal products. This straightforward approach can reduce the mental load often associated with dieting, helping you stay motivated. As you become more familiar with the types of meats that fit within your budget, you will find yourself gaining confidence in your choices, which can significantly bolster your resolve.

When starting out, it's beneficial to set realistic expectations. Weight loss may happen at different rates for each individual, influenced by factors such as metabolism, activity level, and adherence to the diet. Celebrate small milestones along the way, whether it's losing your first few pounds or successfully sticking to your meal plan for a week. Acknowledging these achievements can provide a psychological boost, reinforcing your commitment to the carnivore diet. Remember, each step forward, no matter how small, is a step toward a healthier you.

Challenges are an inevitable part of any dietary change, but they can serve as valuable learning experiences. If you encounter moments of struggle, whether it's cravings for non-carnivore foods or difficulties in sourcing affordable meat options, view these challenges as opportunities to refine your approach. Explore budget-friendly cuts of meat, learn to cook in bulk, and experiment with different recipes to keep your meals enjoyable. This adaptability not only makes the diet more sustainable but also empowers you to overcome obstacles with creativity and resourcefulness.

Lastly, seek community support, whether through online forums, local groups, or social media platforms dedicated to the carnivore diet. Connecting with others who share similar goals can provide motivation and inspiration. Sharing experiences, tips, and even struggles can foster a sense of camaraderie, reminding you that you are not alone on this journey. Embrace the process, stay curious, and remember that every effort you make is a step toward achieving your weight loss goals through the carnivore diet. With determination and the right mindset, you can navigate this journey successfully while keeping your finances in check.

Final Thoughts on the Carnivore Diet and Budgeting

As we conclude this exploration of the carnivore diet and its budget-friendly strategies, it is essential to recognize the unique opportunities this eating plan presents for those seeking weight loss and improved health. The carnivore diet, which emphasizes the consumption of animal products while eliminating carbohydrates, can be both effective and economical with the right approach.

Understanding how to navigate the costs associated with a meat-based diet can empower newcomers to succeed without financial strain, making it a sustainable choice for long-term health.

Budgeting for the carnivore diet begins with proper planning and prioritization. Start by identifying your local meat sources, such as butcher shops, farmers' markets, or wholesale providers, which often offer better prices than conventional grocery stores. Buying in bulk can significantly reduce costs, allowing you to stock up on items like ground beef, chicken thighs, or pork roasts. Additionally, consider options like organ meats, which are nutrient-dense and often less expensive than muscle meats. By diversifying your meat choices and purchasing strategically, you can maintain a satisfying diet while keeping expenses in check.

Transitioning to the carnivore diet can present challenges, particularly for those used to a more varied diet. However, with a focus on budgeting, these challenges can be mitigated. Prepare yourself for potential cravings and the psychological shift that comes from reducing food variety. It may be helpful to establish a simple meal plan that emphasizes your favorite cuts of meat while incorporating affordable options. This not only addresses cravings but also simplifies shopping and cooking, making the transition smoother and more manageable.

Tracking your expenses and progress can also enhance your experience on the carnivore diet. Keep a record of your weekly spending on food, as well as any noticeable changes in your weight and overall well-being. This practice can provide valuable insights into what works best for you, helping you to adjust your strategy as needed. Moreover, celebrating small victories, such as reaching a weight loss milestone or discovering a new favorite recipe, can reinforce your commitment to the diet and encourage you to stick with it.

Ultimately, the carnivore diet can be a viable and budget-conscious approach for those aiming to lose weight and improve their health.

With thoughtful planning, resourcefulness, and a willingness to adapt, beginners can enjoy the benefits of a meat-based diet without enduring financial strain. By implementing effective budgeting strategies and remaining mindful of the challenges, you can successfully navigate your carnivore journey, achieving your goals while savoring the flavors of your new lifestyle.